Breathing
Yourself Thin

Breathing Yourself Thin

Qizhi Gao

Rev. date: 04/22/2017

To order additional copies of this book, contact:
Xlibris
1-888-795-4274
www.Xlibris.com
Orders@Xlibris.com
538247

CONTENTS

Endorsement

You've decided to Change Your Life, Lose Weight, make your Health Priority Number One. This is no easy task, but Dr. Gao will help you attain your goals. I've known Dr. Gao for the past 15 years as my instructor, caregiver, colleague and friend and can attest, first hand, to the results revealed in this book. Why wait? Start your new life now!

Kevin Rieg MD

Acknowledgements

Special thanks to Dr. Loretta Forlaw, PhD, and Dr. Sandra Wilks, DOM, who helped to accomplish this book. As Bigu Qigong instructors, they offered many valuable suggestions. Also thanks to all my Bigu Qigong instructors, Bigu Qigong students, and friends who helped with proofreading and typing. Here is a list of only a few: Tom Overholser, Sandy Evenson, Pam Robinett, Leigh Anne Petersen, Laurinda Wade, Steve Wenke, Madeline Norland, Aliesa George, Bill J. Hawks Jr., Aimon Kopera, Teresa LaCoss, Angela Pottebaum, Jamie Tabor, Yee-Meii Wong, Peggy Case, Nance Tegan and many more. A big thanks to Linda R. Parsons for the final proofreading and editing. And last, I want to thank my lovely wife, Carrie. Without the support and encouragement from her and all my friends, I would not have been able to finish this book.

Introduction

The philosophy of this century is the common sense of the next.
—*from a fortune cookie*

In 1996, I taught a program for Qigong instructors that included both classic and modern Qigong exercises for the purpose of prevention and treatment of disease. At the end of the program, one student said to me, "Dr. Gao, we learned so much on Qigong in this class from common disease to cancer. But we didn't learn how to help weight problems, which more than 50 percent of people are overweight in this country." So I decided to share Bigu Qigong.

Bigu Qigong is a Qigong exercise that harmonizes the mind and regulates breathe with certain body postures to achieve hunger control and improve the function of internal organs. Bigu Qigong is easy to learn and very effective for the goal of achieving and maintaining optimal weight without any side effects.

I conducted my first study of Bigu Qigong on twelve volunteers. The study results were really encouraging, as I expected, and I presented them at the Third World Conference on Medical Qigong in Beijing, China, in 1996. The result was as follows:

> [For the twelve subjects] in the two-week study, there was a significant mean weight loss of 11.2 pounds (5.06 kg) (p<.0001); mean weight loss per day was 0.9 pounds (0.41 kg).[1]

I conducted a second study in 1999.

> At the conclusion of the two-week study, 58 of 74 attended more than 10 classes. There was a . . . mean weight loss of 5.7, 5.69 and 7.66 pounds for . . . subjects from the normal weight group, the overweight group and . . . the obesity group respectively. Even 16 of the 74 who attended only 6 of the classes on the average still lost 2.5, 2.6 and 3.44 pounds, [in each] . . . group respectively.

> The subjects each reported a significant increase in energy levels post exercise for nine of the thirteen days. Hunger levels were significantly reduced ten of thirteen days. Blood pressure did not significantly change between pre- and post-measures.[2]

Weight management classes utilizing Bigu Qigong were offered at my clinic. Class participant results were consistent with study participant results. A local newspaper reported the results for one such class participant in June 1999. The article said, "She lost 18 pounds during the two weeks and continued to lose afterward . . . . She hasn't regained any of the weight."[3]

To date, thousands of people have learned Bigu Qigong through my classes, and the minimum average weight loss was six pounds over the two-week period. Finally, I began to train instructors to meet the demand. During my instructor class, students kept asking me to write

---

[1]   Qizhi Gao, Qigong and Weight Loss, "Qi as a Food Source," in *Third World Conference on Medical Qigong*, (Beijing, China, 1996).

[2]   Qizhi Gao, "Utilizing the Innate Self-Regulatory and Self-Healing Capacity on Weight Management," in *1999 ISSSEEM Conference in Boulder, Co.* (1999).

[3]   *The Wichita Eagle*, "Qigong Takes, Keeps Her Extra Weight off," It Worked for Me, June 29, 1999, main edition, Living Section 1B.

this book. But because of my busy clinic and teaching schedule, I kept putting it off. Finally a deadline presented itself, and I was able to finish the book.

What is the purpose of this book?

The purpose of this book is to *make sense* of weight management, health, and life. When I first arrived in the United States in 1991, I had difficulty speaking or understanding English. One time, a nurse called me on the phone. At the end of the conversation, she asked me, "Does this make sense to you?" I replied, "What means 'Make sense'?" She said, "That means, 'Do you understand?'" I got confused. "I don't understand. That's why I ask you. What is 'Make sense'?" She repeated slowly "'Make sense' means 'understand.'" Since then, I like to use the words *make sense* more than *understand* in my practice and teaching.

We have lots of experts giving us their professional guidance. Most of us trust these recommendations fully but without understanding under what kinds of conditions to follow the suggestions. That is why in many cases you find some famous expert's guidance does not work for you at all. It is wise to think about whether it makes sense or not before you follow it.

For whom do I write this book?

This book is written for the young and the elder—for the person who needs to lose weight, improve health, and have a quality life. This book is for those who wish to take the class, those who wish to teach the class, and those who just want to know more about Bigu Qigong and weight management.

What style of writing will I use for this book?

Originally I was going to write an evidence-based book typical of my profession. And then I found that does not fit my personality. So this book will be a mixture of facts, true personal stories, fables, and some famous words with which you may or may not be familiar.

Life is full of questions, so all chapters will start with a question. I hope you can find an answer. I certainly do not know them all. I just share what I know.

This is not an instruction book. This is a workbook. It requires you to think first to see whether it *makes sense* to you or not. That is your brain exercise. When you read this book, you have to keep your mind open because some of the concepts may be totally new or even strange to you.

Speaking of an open mind, I remember something that happened a number of years ago. I designed an acupuncture treatment plan for a stroke rehabilitation study in a rehabilitation hospital. When I presented my plan to the Institutional Review Board (IRB), a board member expected that I "will get nothing." Upon completion, the study showed that patients who received conventional treatment only (including physical therapy, occupational therapy, speech therapy, and other Western care) experienced a 33 percent discharge to home rate versus a 90 percent discharge to home rate for patients receiving acupuncture plus conventional treatment. That IRB member's response for the positive result was "totally shocked." I replied during the conversation, "You're lucky . . . . You just get shocked. If I take you to China, you will never wake up. You will get a shock, one after the other." He asked me why. I told him that was because we do acupuncture for stroke rehabilitation all the time in China. So keep your mind open; then you will not get shocked later.

If it is true, as the fortune cookie said, "The philosophy of this century is the common sense of the next," then some common sense from two-thousand-year-old Chinese philosophy may shed a bit of light on the subject of weight management and more.

Chapter 1

Why Do You Need to Lose Weight?

Health is the base of life.
—Chinese Proverb

Why do you need to lose weight? This is the first question I ask people who come to me for weight management. The answers are different for each person. Someone may say, "I don't like my appearance." And someone else may say, "My wedding is coming soon, and I try to fit in that wedding gown." The other may say, "I want more energy." These answers are all reasonable but not completely correct.

In traditional Chinese medicine, health means mental, emotional, and physical well-being. From this point of view, your self-esteem, depression, dislike of your appearance, lack of energy, and physical discomfort all belong to the realm of health.

Some people in China use a number system to express happiness. The bigger the number, the happier you are. Each thing that makes you happy is represented by a zero after the number one. For example, if you have a happy family, you add a zero. If you have enough money to make you happy, you add a zero. If you have a talent (like singing), you add a zero. Or if you are smart, you add a zero. Thus, you could become ten, one hundred, one thousand, or ten thousand times happier. But what represents what makes you happy in the first place? No matter how many zeros there are, if you don't have a number one in the first place, the whole thing is zero, which means there must be something that makes you happy that is more important than anything else.

Will your happy family be first? Your money? Your talent? After much debate, you may decide that only your health can occupy the number one position. If you are not healthy, your family will suffer with you. If you are not healthy, you cannot enjoy your money, and you have to spend a lot of your money on medical bills. If you are not healthy, you cannot pursue/perform your talent or use your mental capacity fully. For the Chinese then, health is number one. It is the top priority.

Do you put your health in the top priority? Do you use your resources (time, money, etc.) in that way?

In the United States, we talk about living longer. In China, we talk about living healthy and longer. If you breathe, you have life, but what is the quality of that life? Life and a quality life are completely different. Without health, quality of life diminishes.

So how do we maintain a quality life? By maintaining good health.

We always talk about how busy we are with work, family, or all the things we spend our time on. When they say they are busy, I often ask my patients, "What are you working for?" Lots of them explain using things from the number system. They are working because they love their family or God, they need the money, or they enjoy their talent. I say that is very important, but most important is your health. When you are busy and you don't have time to eat or sleep properly, your health declines. You still have life, but you don't have a good-quality life.

Let me tell you an old Russian story.

To encourage farmers to cultivate virgin land, the empire issued a new policy. It said that a person could own the land for only forty rubles' pay, if that person could run around the perimeter of the land between sunrise and sunset. Farmer Ivan was so excited. He worked hard and dreamed of a rich life. He believed that God gave him this wonderful opportunity to make his dream come true. He was an excellent runner and strong as a horse.

Ivan paid forty rubles. As the sun rose, Ivan started running. He ran toward the east for fifteen miles and then turned south for three miles. He noticed the sun was at its highest. Thirsty and hungry, Ivan started to slow down. He also made up his mind that he wanted the best value for the opportunity. He tried to finish fifteen miles running west and three miles back north to make his perfect rectangle of land, but he was exhausted after nine miles toward the west, and the sun was sinking fast. He decided to use a shortcut back to his starting point. He made it back to the place on time. He ran almost 34 miles that day and earned thirty-six square miles of land, which is 23,040 acres. When the officer come to confirm for Ivan that he was the owner of the land, he was dead from exhaustion.

They buried him on his land—twelve feet by six feet—with his name, Ivan.

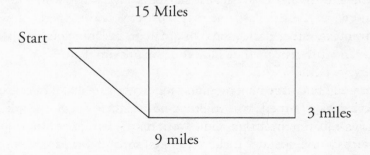

What are you working for? Most of us work to improve our life or living conditions, a house, car, etc. But at what price? Do you want life or quality of life? Why do you need to lose weight? Health, especially by the Chinese definition, is most important. If it does not occupy the number one position, everything else is a zero.

If you agree that your health is the most important thing in your life and that maintaining an optimal weight is good for your health, then you will keep watching your weight (your health) as your highest priority. As a lifelong goal to stay healthy, you will never let your guard down and let your weight bounce up and down.

Chapter 2

How Do You Lose Weight?

Chance favors only the prepared mind.
—Louis Pasteur

As a doctor of Chinese medicine, I respect that the chronic patient is an expert in his/her case because he/she knows what works for him/her and what doesn't. I assume that most of you are experts on weight management, either professional or amateur, because you have already tried many different methods for your weight problem.

All the weight management programs follow the rule that if calorie intake equals calories burned, then there is no weight gain. So people work with this equation in mind. Some work on the left side of the equation to reduce calorie intake, which includes all sorts of diet programs. Some work on the right side of the equation to increase calories burned, which includes different types of physical exercise. Some try programs that work on both sides of the equation. In my weight management classes, I always ask, "What kind of weight management program have you tried?" Here are some typical responses to that question.

Diet Foods:

One recently popular food diet is Atkins. There was a fireman who tried the Atkins diet because he liked meat. It was working, but after six months, he quit because he was tired of meat. He got bored with the diet. His weight returned to its previous level. There are other diets as well that focus on the inclusion or exclusion of one food or type of food or another. Some diets require weighing, counting, or measuring in some fashion. These diets work short-term. However as human beings, we always go back to our normal food, especially when we get sick, tired, bored, or uncomfortable in some way.

Diet Drinks:

There are similar problems with diet drinks. Eating is a social activity. So if you use diet drinks all the time, your life is missing something. Another issue is balance. The drinks say they keep your nutrition balanced, but how can they? Certainly they include many of the nutrients that we know to be necessary for health and wellness, but they do not (cannot) include all the things in normal food. For example, there is vitamin C in tomatoes and a diet drink may include vitamin C as an essential nutrient. However, what else is in tomatoes that your body needs that modern science has not yet discovered? New discoveries are made all the time.

Diet Pills:

I have seen many problems with this method. Diet pills are often a cover for laziness. People want a magic pill. They think you can just put one in your mouth, and it will curb your appetite and you lose weight. The pills give you the wrong signal. You don't have to work at all; you just pop a couple of pills. Most often, your weight will go up and down several times, which in turn causes you to age faster and creates wrinkles.

Weight Lifting or Other Exercises:

Lots of people are talking about exercise. Exercise is good, according to the equation. If you do more and eat less, you will lose weight. The problem is time and energy. Between your work and your family, you don't have that much time and energy to exercise. You are already exhausted. Then on top of that, you try to add on another hour for exercise. Lots of people come to my clinic and tell me they're so tired from work and family that they skip exercise. They skip once or twice or three times, and pretty soon, they just go ahead and buy a bigger size of clothes. This seems to be especially true from October through December, when people will put on that extra ten to fifteen pounds. So weight lifting or physical exercise is always good for you. It's just whether you have the ability, time, or energy to do it.

One time I even heard of a person who wore some sort of *plastic coat, sweating, while walking*. People really do a lot of work to lose weight!

In short, all these methods work in the short term. I'm not saying they're not good, but they just don't last. Why?

I believe that goal setting is the key.

How much weight you need to lose is just a number. When you reach that number, you let your guard down. Then before you know, the weight, or even more, is put right back on.

The goal for weight management is not just the number of pounds or inches you want to lose. The goal is to improve your health. If you put your health in the top priority, you will never let your guard down.

What is the healthy, affordable, and easy way to lose weight and keep the weight off? Let's see whether Bigu Qigong is a fit for you.

Chapter 3

What is Bigu Qigong?

Definition, History, and Personal Notes

Qigong is that practice the vital energy makes you stay in a perfect health state.
—Qizhi Gao

What is the meaning of *Bigu*?
bi (pronounced *bee*)—avoid
gu (pronounced *goo*)—grain

What is the meaning of *Qigong?*
qi (pronounced *chee*)—vital energy
gong (pronounced *kung*)—kung fu

Kung fu means that practice makes perfect. A tailor is the kung fu master of making clothes. A carpenter is the kung fu master of building a house or making furniture. Qigong has thousands of different forms for different purposes. In ancient times, Qigong (or Daoyin as it was more commonly called then) was used for health improvement and for martial arts combat. Daoyin means leading (the qi or vital energy) to someplace. In this context, it means guiding your energy deep inside your body for health. Simply speaking, Qigong means practice your vital energy to keep you in a perfect physical and mental state.

Bigu Qigong harmonizes the mind: breathe while in certain body postures to achieve hunger control and to improve the functioning of inner organs for the goal of optimal weight and health. Bigu Qigong has three key elements, as do other Qigong exercises: mind, breath, and body posture. By harmonizing the mind, regulating breathe, and adjusting body posture, Bigu Qigong achieves hunger control and improves the functioning of inner organs for the goal of optimal weight and health.

Bigu is a Qigong phenomenon. If Qigong practitioners practice Qigong to a certain level, they don't rely on food and can live for a period of time without food. They use this period of time to purify their body energy. Bigu can be found in many ancient Chinese texts, in individual legends, and in exercise methods. Here are a few examples.

Among the historic relics unearthed from Han tomb number 3 at Mawangdui, Changsha, Hunan Province, there was a silk book, *On Abandoning Food and Living on Qi,* and a silk painting, *Daoyin Illustrations*, of the early Western Han dynasty period (third century BC). The former is a method of "inducing, promoting, and conducting qi"; the latter displays forty-four colored *Daoyin Illustrations* in which training exercises are painted.

Wang Chong *Lun Heng—Dao Xue Pian* from the Eastern Han dynasty (25–220 BC), stated, "The people who live on qi have longevity. Although they do not eat enough grain, they are still full of energy."

A story from *Bao Puzi's Inner Treaties* said that a man named Jian was hunting in the field when he fell into a deep tomb. He could not climb out. He was so hungry. Then he saw a big turtle. Its head moved up and down to swallow the air. Jian had been told that a turtle is good at Daoyin (that is, good at conducting qi). He imitated the turtle's movement. He did not feel hungry anymore until someone saved him one hundred days later. After that, he had the Bigu ability—living on the air without food. Emperor Wei did not believe this and placed Jian in a room without food. One year later, Jian was still full of energy and his face had a normal, healthy color. The emperor finally set him free.

One more word is *breatharian*. Omnivores consume meat and plant food, water, and air. Carnivores consume only meat food, water, and air. Herbivores, or vegetarians, consume only plant food, water, and air. Breatharians, on the other hand, consume only what comes to them in the air they breathe, thus the name "*breath*arian."

As a Qigong practitioner, I have personally experienced Bigu twice. From July 20, 1995, until August 3, 1995, my daily diet consisted of a cup of juice or an orange. The first three days were the most diffcult as I continued to feel hungry. After the three-day adjustment period, I was able to control my appetite and hunger with the Qigong exercise and gradually increased my energy level as well. I continued my normal daily work routine during the two-week period and required less sleep than normal. Physically and mentally, I felt very comfortable and relaxed. I lost a total of fifteen pounds in two weeks and have never gained the weight back. I repeated the same process for a two-week period in 1996 with similar results.

The most important points need to be clear here. Bigu is a Qigong phenomenon. Bigu Qigong is the name of the Qigong exercise for the purpose of weight management. Bigu Qigong is not to teach fasting.

It has two rules to follow. They are the following: (1) eat only when you are hungry, and (2) drink only when you are thirsty. These two rules mean we never encourage any student to fast or to drink/not drink.

Eat only when you are hungry; drink only when you are thirsty.

For the people who want to lose weight, most of them understand the first rule. But I often get challenged on the second rule, "Drink only when you are thirsty." We have been told for a long time now to drink eight glasses of water a day to eliminate toxins from our body. Since 1996, I have explained the second rule to all my weight management classes from three different aspects.

First, let us look at our body structure. Our body is not designed with different pockets, some of which holding minerals, nutrients, or vitamins—the good stuff the body needs—and others holding toxins—the bad stuff the body needs to get rid of. So, the brain would have a hard time to figure out which pockets need to be flushed out. If we drink more than we need to, we will dilute all the good stuff and bad stuff and flush them all out together, right? This is the first reason I disagree with the rule of drinking eight glasses of water a day.

The second reason is that it is not scientific to drink eight glasses of water a day without considering age, sex, and profession. Do you think fifteen-year-olds and seventy-five-year-olds need to drink the same amount of water a day? Do you think a doctor working indoors and a farmer working in a field under the sun should consume the same amount of water?

The third reason I disagree is that it is harmful. If your body doesn't need eight glasses of water a day, and you force yourself to drink them, the extra fluid has to be expelled. What does that job? Your kidneys and bladder have to. They have to do extra work to expel the extra fluid. After a period of time, your kidneys and bladder will wear out and frequent urination, incontinence, or difficulty passing urine will be the result.

Consider. An astronomer was excited about the stars in the sky and did not pay attention to the ground. He fell into a well. He yelled for help. Someone went to rescue him and learned what had happened to him. The rescuer said, "Science without common sense could be dangerous."

So eat only when you're hungry and drink only when you're thirsty. These are the golden rules for your weight management.

Bigu Qigong is not fasting. It is safe if you follow the rules (see studies in chapter 9). Thousands have employed Bigu Qigong with no complaints or side effects, including those with stomach problems and diabetes. It will improve your whole body and not just help you lose weight.

The ancient Chinese philosophy of yin, yang, and the five elements has guided Chinese medicine for the last two thousand years. If the fortune cookie is correct, this is the common sense for our time.

Chapter 4

How Do You Do Bigu Qigong?

Practice makes perfect.
—Chinese Proverb

Bigu Qigong consists of two parts. Part 1, Frog Qigong, is an exercise to control appetite. Part 2, Lotus Sitting, is an exercise to retain energy.

Self-massage is also highly recommended.

Each is explained below.

Part 1: Frog Qigong

Frog Qigong consists of three elements: preparation, main exercise, and closure.

Preparation

Sit in a chair. Place feet flat on the floor, with the thigh and the calf in an approximate ninety-degree angle. Posture is straight and the back is not touching the chair's back. Relax your body (Picture 1). Place your tongue on the roof of your mouth, right behind the teeth. Close your eyes slightly. Think of something positive. Inhale through your nose and exhale through your mouth three times.

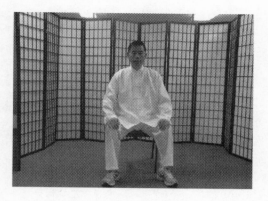

Picture 1

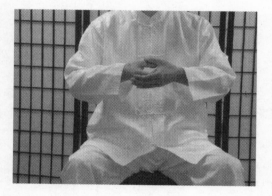

Picture 2

Then place your hands as shown in Picture 2. Men place hands exactly as in Picture 2 with the left fingers wrapping around the right. Women wrap right fingers around the left. Rest your elbows on top of your knees (Picture 3). Then lay your head on top of your hands (Picture 4).

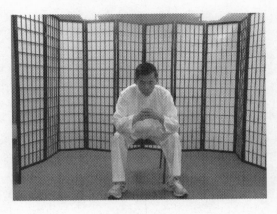

Picture 3

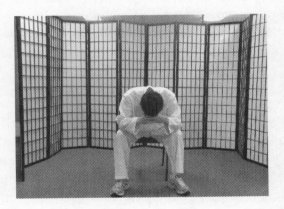

Picture 4

Inhale naturally through your nose, and exhale through your mouth three more times. This will expel all the turbid energy or impure air from your lungs.

Main exercise

Retain the posture shown in Picture 4. Do the following exercise for fifteen minutes. Inhale through your nose to 30 percent of your normal lung capacity. Stop. Say a positive word in your mind, *not* out loud. For example, you might say *peaceful, harmony,* or *healthy.* Any word you choose is fine; just choose a word and don't change it. Inhale another 40 percent. Then exhale fully, *all through your nose.*

Let me repeat. Breathe in the following pattern for the entire fifteen minutes:

Inhale to 30 percent capacity and stop. Speak the word in your mind. Inhale another 40 percent. Exhale fully. Notice that you are only inhaling to 70 percent of your full capacity. If you force yourself to inhale to full capacity in that position, you will have sore ribs. I don't want anyone to complain about that!

It is not necessary to set a timer or watch the clock. In fact, you should not watch a clock. You can count your breaths. Normally, a healthy person will breathe ten to fifteen times a minute. On the average, then, two hundred breaths would be close to fifteen minutes. If you breathe deeply or after you have practiced for a while, 150 breaths are more likely. You will come to know about how many breaths is fifteen minutes for you.

Closure

Return to normal breathing with your eyes still closed. From the position in Picture 4, raise your head slowly. Rub your hands together until you feel warm (Picture 5). Place your hands on your face (Picture 6). Massage as if you were washing your face ten to twenty times (Picture 7). Slowly open your eyes. Stand and stretch. This completes the exercise.

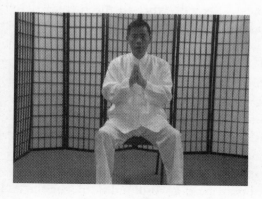

Picture 5

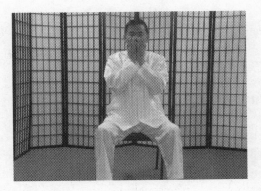

Picture 6

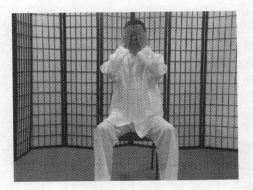

Picture 7

Most people who lose ten or fifteen pounds in two weeks have poor skin color and become wrinkled in the face. In our exercise, sitting in the forward position and massaging the face at the end each time will reduce or eliminate these effects. The forward position places the head at or below heart level, which lets blood go to the brain/head more readily. The face is nourished by the blood flow. The massage also encourages circulation. So after you do the exercise, even in your first fifteen-minute try, you will feel so relaxed and your mind so clear. After two weeks in my class, most people who lost more than six pound and even those who lost fifteen to twenty pounds, still had healthy color and firm skin on their face. This is a healthy weight loss. You will never have that exhausted, sick look.

This exercise should be done one hour before each meal for the best results. And you have to follow the two rules:

www.ibreathin.com

Eat when you are hungry.

Drink when you are thirsty.

Part 2: Lotus Sitting

This exercise is fairly simple, but it requires a lot of concentration. First, sit comfortably. Slowly close your eyes. Keep your mind focused. Relax. Place your tongue on your upper palate right behind your teeth. Slowly place your hands together with fingertips touching like you're holding a ball in your hands (Picture 8). Put this ball on your belly button with half of the ball inside your tummy and the other half in your hands. Allow some space between your arms and your sides. The correct position is shown in Picture 9; the incorrect (with arms tight against your sides), is Picture 10.

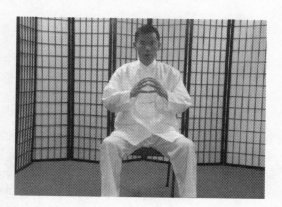

Picture 8

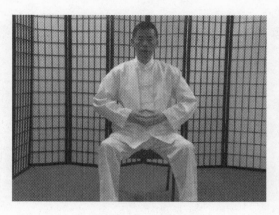

Picture 9 (correct sitting)

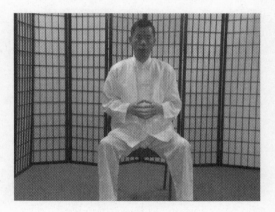

Picture 10 (incorrect sitting)

Using the position in Picture 9, inhale so that the air goes into your chest. Your chest expands and your tummy goes back (Picture 11–14). When you exhale, let the air go out freely. This is different from your normal breathing. Breathe in this manner for ten to fifteen minutes.

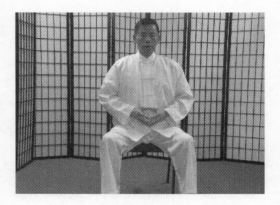

Picture 11 (breathe in)

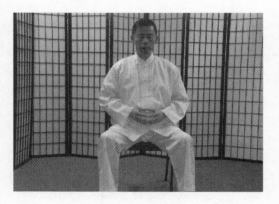

Picture 12 (breathe out)

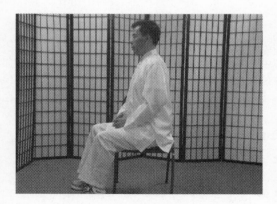

Picture 13 (breathe in)

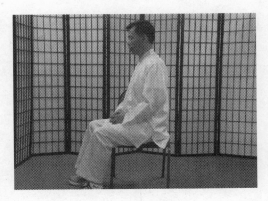

Picture 14 (breathe out)

After ten to fifteen minutes, slowly put your hands together, covering your belly button. For men, the left hand touches the belly button and the right hand is on top (Picture 15). For women, the right hand touches the belly button with the left hand on top. From this position, move your hands counterclockwise (to the left). Make nine circles, starting small and getting bigger. The biggest of the nine circles will *not* go up past your sternum (breastbone) or down past your pubic bone. The circles will *not* go left or right past the side of your body (Picture 16). Then you will make nine circles, moving your hands clockwise, from big to small, ending where you began—centered on the belly button. Breathe normally during the time that you are making the circles with your hands.

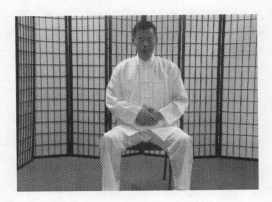

Picture 15

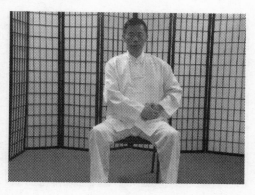

Picture 16

Your eyes should remain closed throughout all of Part 2: Lotus Sitting. Open them slowly after completing the circles. You may also do this exercise seated in the lotus position on the floor. Use the same hand positions and breathing routine. This exercise should be done at least once a day. For people with a weak constitution or chronic fatigue, it is highly recommended that they do this exercise twice a day, morning and evening.

Self-Massage

It is highly recommended that self-massage follow the Bigu Qigong exercise. This self-massage technique may also improve your health and prevent disease even when you are not doing Bigu Qigong. It has a long history of promoting anti-aging and self-healing. It is simple to learn. Each massage movement provides its own health benefit. Each movement and its associated benefit follows.

To begin, relax your body in a sitting position (Picture 17).

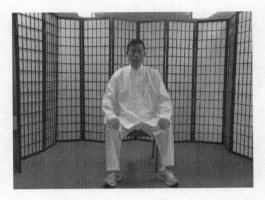

Picture 17

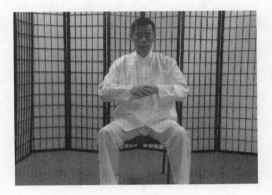

Picture 18

1. Hands: Place your right palm on top of your left hand. Move your right hand up and down the length of your left hand, from fingertips to the wrist and back (Picture 18). This is one repetition. Do nine repetitions. Switch your hands and do nine repetitions with your left hand on top of your right. From a Western point of view, this movement is good for rheumatoid arthritis and peripheral neuropathy in your hands, carpal tunnel syndrome, and Raynaud's disease. In Chinese medicine, the hand relates to six meridians, which are the lung, the heart, the pericardium, the large intestine, the small intestine, and the triple warmer; so massaging our hands will stimulate six meridians of the body. This will have more effects than just the few I've mentioned.

2. Arm and shoulder: Place your right palm on your left arm at the wrist. Massage on the inside of the arm, going up, around the shoulder, and down the outside of the arm (Pictures 19–22). This is one repetition. Do nine repetitions. Switch your hands and do nine repetitions with your left hand on your right arm. This movement is good for rheumatoid arthritis that causes elbow pain, carpal tunnel syndrome, tennis elbow, and frozen shoulder.

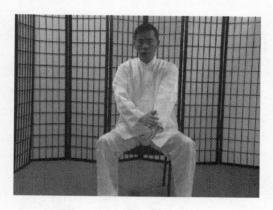

Picture 19

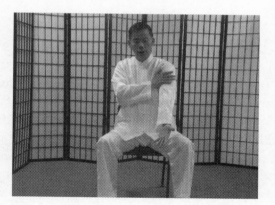

Picture 20

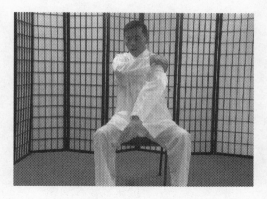

Picture 21

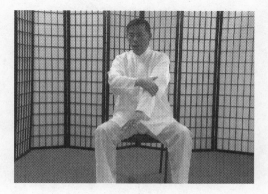

Picture 22

3. Eye: Place your thumbs (Picture 23) on your temples (Picture 24). Using the middle section of your index finger (Picture 25), massage your eyebrow from inside to outside, and then massage the lower orbit of the eye in the same manner (Picture 26). This is one repetition. Do nine repetitions. The thumbs remain in contact with your temples throughout this section. The pressure point there will help with migraine headaches. The eye socket massage helps with nearsightedness, farsightedness, and night blindness and helps prevent eye-related diseases.

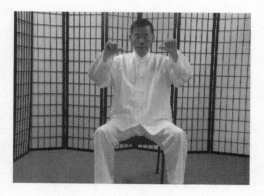

Picture 23

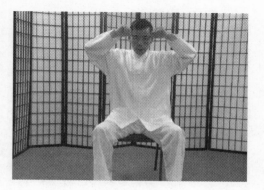

Picture 24

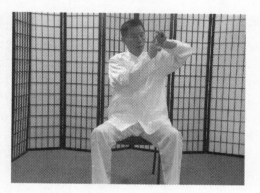

Picture 25

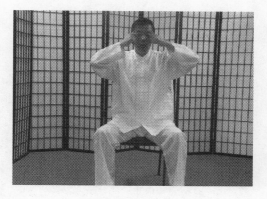

Picture 26

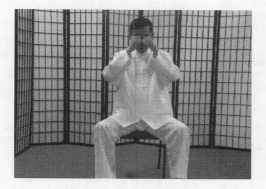

Picture 27

4. Inner canthus: Place your thumbs on the inner canthus—
   that is, on either side of the bridge of your nose, next to the
   eyes (Picture 27). Make nine circles with your thumbs in one
   direction and then nine circles in the other direction (Picture
   28). This movement is good for dry eyes, itchy eyes, burning
   eyes, blurred vision, and eye-related diseases.

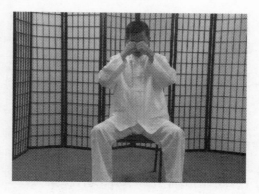

Picture 28

5. Bridge of nose: Place the thumb and the index finger of your right hand across the bridge of your nose by your eyes, and place your left hand on the back of your head (Pictures 29 and 30). Gently pinch the bridge of your nose and release (by pulling your hand away from your nose) while, at the same time, moving your other hand down the back of your head (Picture 31). Do this nine times. Switch hands and do nine repetitions. This is good for dry eyes, itchy eyes, burning eyes, sinus, and allergies.

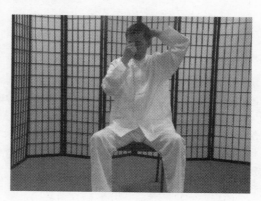

Picture 29

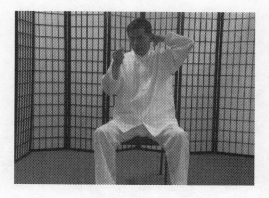

Picture 30

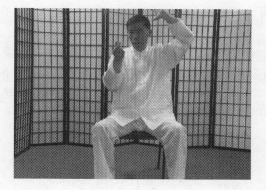

Picture 31

6. Nose: Place your index fingers on either side of your nose by the nostrils (Picture 32). Move your fingers up and down along the side of the nose. This is one repetition. Do thirty-six repetitions. This is good for sinus problems, allergies, and preventing colds and flu.

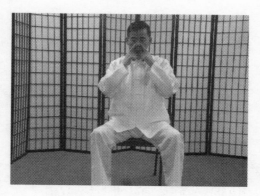

Pictures 32

7. Beat the drum: Cover your ears as shown (Picture 33) and tap ("beat") the back of your head with your fingers several times (Picture 34). Apply slight pressure to your ears and then pull your hands away. This is one repetition. Do nine repetitions. This is good for dizziness, tinnitus (ringing in the ears), hearing loss, and other hearing-related diseases.

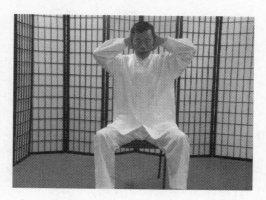

Pictures 33

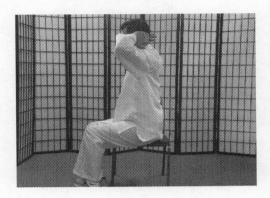

Pictures 34

8. Unplug the ear: Place the tips of both index fingers in the ears (Picture 35), twist the hands back and forth, and then with a slightly forward, flicking motion, pull them out (Picture 36). This is one repetition. Do nine repetitions. This is good for dizziness, tinnitus, hearing loss, and other ear-related diseases.

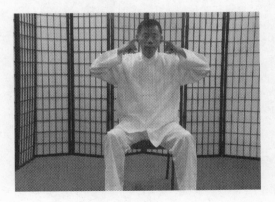

Picture 35

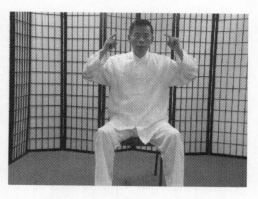

Picture 36

9. Click teeth. With your lips closed, click your upper and lower teeth together (Picture 37). Do this thirty-six times. This is good for preventing toothache and other tooth-related diseases.

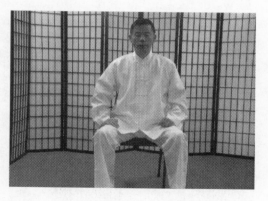

Picture 37

10. Tongue: Rotate your tongue in your mouth to generate more saliva. Rotate until your mouth is full of saliva. Then, swallow the saliva in three portions (one-third each swallow). This is good for dry mouth, weak constitution, and other digestive-related diseases.

11. Dry face wash: Place your hands on your face then, starting at your chin, massage upward by your nose to your forehead (Pictures 38 and 39). At the forehead, move hands out slightly and come down the cheeks/side of the face. This is one repetition. Do nine repetitions. This will help you look younger.

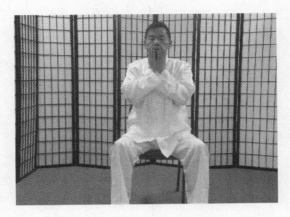

Picture 38

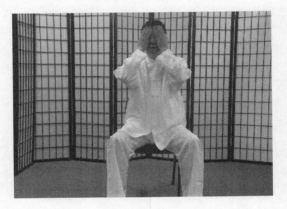

Picture 39

12. Head: Use your ten fingers to make ten lines in your hair from the forehead to the back of the head (Pictures 40 and 41). Go all the way back and down to the base of the skull. This is one repetition. Do nine repetitions. This will help lower blood pressure and help relieve headaches, insomnia, and listlessness.

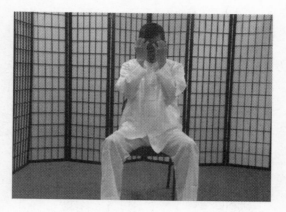

Picture 40

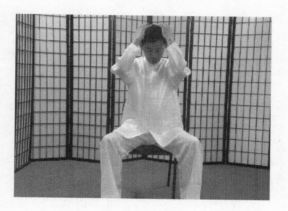

Picture 41

13. Chest: Begin by placing your right hand on your upper right chest (Picture 42). Move your hand diagonally across and down to end as in Picture 43. Do the same movement with your left hand (Pictures 44 and 45). This is one repetition. Do nine repetitions. This movement is good for depression, fluid retention, acid reflux, heartburn, and other digestive-related diseases.

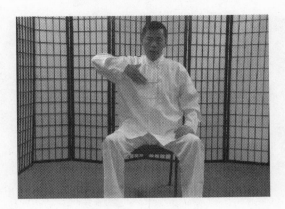

Picture 42

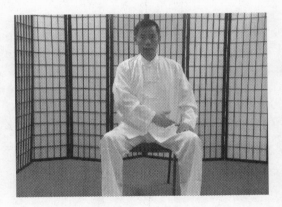

Picture 43

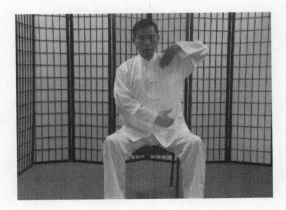

Picture 44

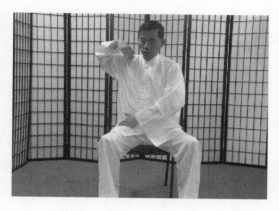

Picture 45

14. Abdomen: Place your right hand on your belly button and make nine clockwise circles on your abdomen. Then, place your left hand on your belly button and make nine counterclockwise circles. This is good for abdominal distention, diarrhea, constipation, and other gastrointestinal tract-related diseases. For constipation, do *only* the clockwise direction. For diarrhea, do *only* the counterclockwise direction (Pictures 46 and 47).

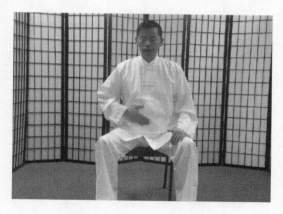

Picture 46

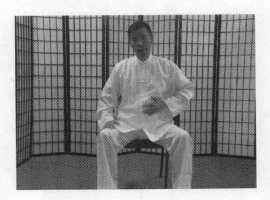

Picture 47

15. Back: Place both hands on your back and massage up and down. Begin as in Picture 48, move to Picture 49, and come back down. This is one repetition. Do at least thirty-six repetitions. This is good for low back pain, sciatic nerve pain, diarrhea, constipation, and some kidney-related diseases.

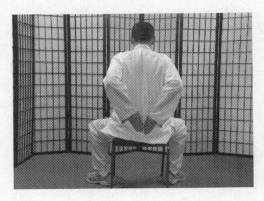

Picture 48

16. Leg: Put both of your hands on the upper left leg (Picture 50). Slowly push down to the ankle (Picture 51) then pull back up. This is one repetition. Do nine repetitions. Repeat the same process with both hands on the right leg (Pictures 52 and 53). This is good for leg pain, sciatic pain, knee pain, or knee weakness.

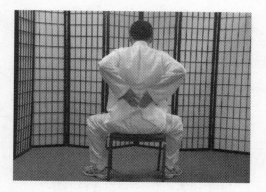

Picture 49

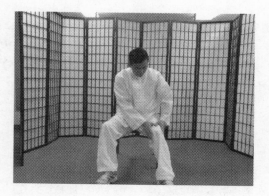

Picture 50

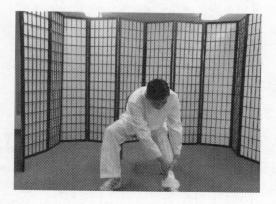

Picture 51

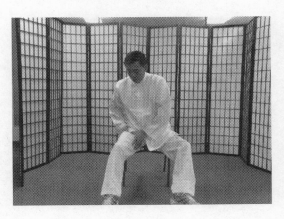

Picture 52

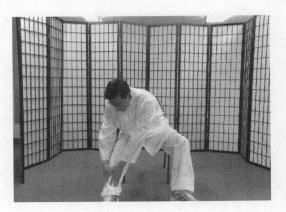

Picture 53

17. Knee: Put both hands on your knees. Your left palm will cover your left knee; your right palm will cover your right knee. Massage your knees in small circles with your left hand moving clockwise and your right hand moving counterclockwise (Pictures 54–56). Make nine circles. Then reverse the direction of the circles. Do nine circles with your left hand moving counterclockwise and your right hand moving clockwise. This is good for knee pain or knee weakness. In Chinese medicine, we say you age from the leg. If you have knee pain or knee weakness, it shows you are aging. So doing more of this part will help you to walk more and live longer.

QIZHI GAO

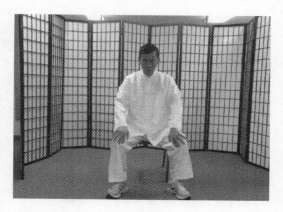

Picture 54

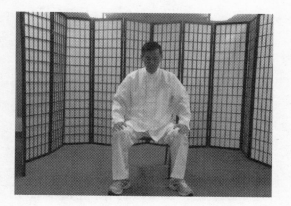

Picture 55

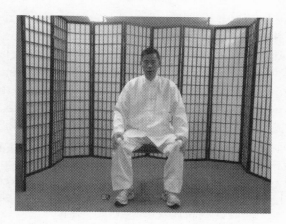

Picture 56

18. Feet: Use the palm of your right hand to rub the bottom of
    your left foot in a slight diagonal movement. (Place left foot
    on right leg without shoes, as shown.) Move your hand up and
    down (Pictures 57 and 58). This is one repetition. Do thirty-
    six repetitions. Repeat the same process with the left hand on
    the right foot. Remember, in Chinese medicine, aging starts
    in the legs. If your feet cannot walk, your legs are useless. So
    protecting your feet is very important. That is why you have
    to do thirty-six repetitions. This is good for foot pain, chronic
    fatigue, and peripheral neuropathy of the feet.

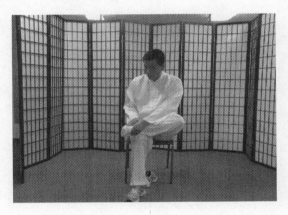

Picture 57

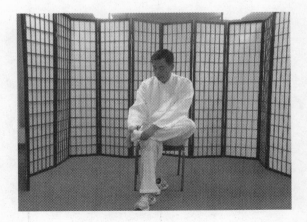

Picture 58

Self-massage can be tailored to your personal needs. If you have a knee problem, then massage your knees more. You can do self-massage anytime you want to, even when you watch TV. The number of repetitions recommended for each part of the body are just to help beginners learn the massage. You can do more repetitions if your body needs them.

Chapter 5

How Does Bigu Qigong Work?

Eastern and Western Theories of Weight Loss

You will never lose a battle if you know yourself and your counterpart well enough.
—*Sunzi*

Recall from chapter 2 that in Western medicine, weight management programs follow the rule that there is no weight gain if calorie intake equals calories burned. Chinese medicine believes that everybody is different, so it is not enough to simply follow the rule. For example, you and your sisters/brothers sit at the same table, eating the same food, and your sisters/brothers are even less diligent about physical exercise. You gain weight, and the others do not. Sometimes it seems that even if you have nothing but water, you still gain weight. Somehow, you are different. More and more Western weight management programs *now* not only follow the rule, but are also starting to recognize that individuals are different. Hence, it is no longer enough to only talk about how much you eat and how much exercise you do. What's going on inside your body also plays a very important role. Western weight management programs address this with behavior modification and lifestyle changes but seldom mention the difference among individuals.

Bigu Qigong exercise covers all these aspects: appetite control, physical exercise, and behavior modification or lifestyle changes. The difference among individuals is also considered as an important part for the success of the program.

What is the difference among individuals? Simply speaking, it related to the function of one's internal organs. If your internal organs work properly and harmonize together, then you should have a healthy body. As I mentioned in chapter 1, weight issues are health issues. The internal organs' dysfunction, in most cases, could be a cause or a result of weight gain.

Now, let us see how Bigu Qigong controls appetite, improves internal organs' function, and conserves energy to achieve healthy and optimal weight.

Bigu Qigong exercise will help you to improve the functioning of your internal organs by making your diaphragm go up and down much farther than the normal range. This is physical exercise on the inside of your body and is different from the physical exercise you get when you go to the gym. At the gym, you consume your physical energy. In Bigu Qigong, you conserve your energy. This is a big difference.

Bigu Qigong consists of two parts. Part 1 is Frog Qigong. Part 2 is Lotus Sitting. How to do these is explained in chapter 4. Here we will discuss the theory.

In Part 1, Frog Qigong,

1. The body position (Picture 59) places the head at or below heart level, which helps the blood flow to the head and the face more readily. It improves the brain function and keeps facial color healthy and the skin firm even when you've lost ten to twenty pounds in a short period of time.
2. The breathing pattern causes the diaphragm to move up and down in a wider range, which
   (a) produces the fullness in the chest that reduces the hungry feeling and

(a) gently massages the organs in your lower abdominal cavity to make internal organs function better.

Frog Qigong stimulates all bodily functions and utilizes body fat as an energy source. Hunger and food intake are minimized and weight loss is realized. Facial wrinkles generally experienced during weight loss are minimized, and skin luster is retained.

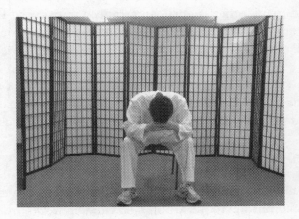

Picture 59

Part 2, Lotus Sitting, is a modified version of a classic Qigong exercise that helps conserve energy to compensate for decreased energy from less food intake.

Here is an example to help make sense of Bigu Qigong and the difference between Bigu Qigong and physical exercise.

One student, who is a medical doctor, had done four months in a boot camp. He was up every morning early to do the push-ups, running, etc., required of him. He did not lose any weight in that four-month period. In two weeks of the weight management class utilizing Bigu Qigong, he lost over fourteen pounds. He was really mad because he had worked so hard without losing anything until he came to the class. Perhaps clearer: This tells you his body had been working too hard. All the calories he took in while in boot camp were used to fuel/maintain his exhaustion. With the Bigu Qigong exercise, he conserved his energy and improved the function of his internal organs. This allowed him to lose weight. The calorie rule doesn't work if all you're doing is using the calories to maintain your exhaustion from overdoing physical exercise.

In Chinese medicine, your digestion is controlled by your internal organs working in harmony. It's not just your stomach or intestines; digestion is also related to your other organs. For example, liver enzymes, the spleen, and bile from the gallbladder all play important roles. Stress, fatigue, and many other factors can seriously impact the functioning of your system. Poor functioning results in a lack of harmony and poor digestion. Poor digestion results in weight management problems.

It is a behavior modification and lifestyle change for most of us to do Bigu Qigong daily and consistently. You have to do the exercise to get the result. If you don't do the exercise, there is no free lunch.

To summarize, from a Western point of view Bigu Qigong works by addressing the anatomy and physiology (via body position and breathing) and psychology (via the discipline) necessary to produce weight loss. From an Eastern point of view, it works by addressing energy flow to create improved function of internal organs and the harmony of mind, breath, and body necessary for weight management.

Chapter 6

Why Bigu Qigong?

It is not the answer that enlightens, but the question.
—*Eugene Lonesco*

Bigu Qigong includes all the elements necessary for success—food intake reduction, exercise, and mental discipline—without the pitfalls of the usual Western weight management programs. It can be practiced independently as a weight loss program. It can also work *with* any other weight management program.

In chapter 2, we discussed diet food, diet drinks, diet pills, weight lifting, and other physical exercises. All these will work short-term, but each has pitfalls or drawbacks. Bigu Qigong has

- no physical limitation (as long as you can sit or lie down comfortably);
- no drug or pill use;
- no food limitation;
- no weighing, measuring, or counting;
- no strenuous exercise; and
- no side effects

and it

- is easy to learn,
- has quick-to-see results, and
- promotes overall health improvement.

The difficulty with Bigu Qigong is the same as with every other management program. It won't work if you don't do it.

Here is a short story.

A farmer was working in the field on a hot day when he saw a rabbit run into a tree. The farmer caught the rabbit and made a delicious dinner. Compared with the hard work in the field, the farmer decided to wait under the tree for the next rabbit. Time passed by. The farmer lost his growing season and never found another bad luck rabbit.

Are we better than that farmer? For weight management, are we looking for a "magic bullet" (pill, food, drink) that will let us lose weight without effort? Why not manage your weight in a way that works with your body, with no side effects and no additional costs once you learn it? Why *not* do Bigu Qigong?

Chapter 7

How Do You Get the Best
Results from Bigu Qigong?

Concentration, Correction, and Consistency

There is no free lunch.
—Wise Man

You will get the best results from Bigu Qigong by using the three Cs: concentration, correction, and consistency.

Concentration: If you are doing the exercise and your mind is not there, you won't get the result. Concentrate on the exercise and nothing else.

Correction: Check and correct your mind, breathing, and body posture every time.

Consistency: If you do the exercise only when you feel like it, you won't get the result. There is no free lunch.

A few stories will illustrate these points.

Educated Lady

A well-educated lady with good health consciousness came to see me for her health concerns. She said she started doing (transcendental) meditation in the 1970s and was expecting the health benefits of that practice. She asked, "Why am I still getting sick?" I asked her how she did the exercise.

She said she sat in the same place at the same time every day. It was quiet. In a calm state, she prayed for her husband's business and for the kids; she checked what she did right and what she did wrong. I told her, "That's not transcendental meditation. Transcendental meditation is when you are in a state in which you don't know who you are or where you are. You don't consciously think about anything. In other words, you never enter the "transcendental state." What you are doing is having a quiet time to sort out your life. You did not do the exercise correctly. That's why even though you've been doing this for thirty or forty years, you don't have the result."

She had great consistency but did not concentrate on the exercise or check that she was doing the exercise correctly.

Kitten fishing

A mother cat took her kitten to fish. The little kitten threw the fishhook in the water. He watched and waited for the float to sink, which, his mom told him, means a fish bit the hook. He watched and waited, watched and waited. The float moved back and forth, from left to right, but never sank.

A butterfly came and flew around. The little kitten saw the butterfly. He put down his fishing pole and tried to catch the butterfly. The butterfly flew away. Disappointed, the little kitten went back to the mother cat. "Mother, you got a fish!" yelled the little kitten in surprise. "You will get one too, baby, if you sit there and fish." The little kitten mumbled, "I was sitting there fishing, but no fish bit." The little kitten sat down to watch the float again. He watched and waited, watched and waited. The float moved back and forth, from left to the right, but never sank.

A dragonfly came and flew around. The little kitten saw the dragonfly. He put down his fishing pole and tried to catch the dragonfly. The dragonfly flew away. Disappointed, the little kitten went back to the mother cat. "Mother, you got another fish!" yelled the little kitten in surprise. The mother cat said, "You have to pay attention to what you are doing, then you will get a fish. If you cannot focus on what you are doing, you will never get a fish."

Can you get the fish? If you change your goal all the time, then you cannot get anything. For your weight management, concentrate on your goal. Remember, your ultimate goal is your health.

We are all bothered by regular life. Things happen that tempt us to focus on something of lesser importance. If your health is in the number one position, as we discussed in chapter 1, then that must be what you concentrate on rather than other things. Concentrate on your goal.

Village man

An old man lived with his sixteen-year-old son in a village. The village was between two countries, and a horse was the only property he owned. One day, the horse ran away. Village people went to comfort him. The old man said, "Please don't worry about me. Maybe the loss is not a bad thing." A few days later, the horse came back and brought a herd of cattle. Suddenly the old man became rich, and the village people went to congratulate him. The old man said, "Please don't be so happy. Maybe some bad thing will happen." Just like he said, a few days later, his son fell off the horse and broke his leg. The matchmakers stopped visiting the newly rich village man because no girl wanted to marry the son, whose leg was broken. To reply to the sympathy from the village people, the old man said, "Lucky may come after the unlucky." Not very long after, a war happened between the two countries, and all the men were required to join the army. Nine out of ten died on the battlefield. The limping young man became popular again.

The moral of the story is that happiness may lead to unhappiness and bad luck may lead to good luck. Keep a peaceful mind and strive for harmony.

Concentration requires a peaceful mind.

Nine-yard Alley

Once upon a time, two rich men lived as neighbors. There was a five-yard-wide alley between the two neighbors' houses. One day, one of the neighbors started to remodel his house. He decided to move the wall over one yard to make his front yard bigger. The other neighbor wanted his bigger too. He did the same thing his neighbor had done. This made the five-yard-wide alley only three yards wide. This was a problem. Everybody complained because the road was too narrow for the coach to go through. Neither of the neighbors wanted to back off their newly built wall. The arguments started and then a lawsuit was filed. The judge knew what to do, but he didn't want to do it because the prime minister was the brother of the one who started it. The case was unsettled for over a year.

Finally, the first rich man decided to write a letter to his brother, asking for a favor to settle the case. In the reply the prime minister said, "Dear brother: With all of your land and money, why do you care about one yard of the alley? It would embarrass your neighbor if you back off three yards to show how generous you are." So the young brother did. The neighbor heard the story and thought, *I have the same wealth as my neighbor, and I am a generous man too.* So he backed off three yards also. The case was solved with a nine-yard alley.

In our daily life, arguments among family members and competition among businesses happen all the time. The moral of this story is that tolerance makes peace, and harmony makes prosperity. Then, you can concentrate on your health and enjoy life more.

Farmer and his Crop

A farmer thought his crop grew too slowly as compared to his neighbor's crop. He thought he would help it. He pulled all the plants up an inch higher. What did he see next? The crops were all dead. It is very important to follow natural law. You must go step by step. In any weight management program, do not expect overnight change. Steady, stable progress is best. Be consistent in your practice. Do not change your goal. Your goal is for health.

The Knot in the Yo-Yo's String

The yo-yo was a popular toy when my son, Daniel, was eight years old. He loved to play with it but often came to me for help because there was a knot in the yo-yo's string. One day, I untied the knot for him and showed him how to untie it. A few minutes later, he came back for the same reason. After a few times of repeating this process, I decided to put my work down and help him solve the problem.

I sat down with him and showed him again how to untie the knot. Then I tied the knot back in the string. He looked at me in surprise. "Dad, you tied a knot in the string!" "Yes, do you need more to practice?" While I replied, I tied another knot. He realized that now he had to untie these knots. He tried and soon got frustrated. "There was just one knot in the string when I came to you for help, now I've got two," he complained. I asked, "Do you need more to practice?" I tied another knot in the string. He got really mad at me. "Dad! I am going to cut this one off and get a new string." I said, "That is exactly what many adults have done or will do when they encounter some frustrating thing or task. That is, they give up this one and get another one." He looked at me with a puzzled expression.

Will you decide, "If I don't like this, I'll just do something else"? Or will you stick to your goal, practice consistently, concentrate when you do the exercise, and make sure that you do it correctly? Bigu Qigong will work, and you can achieve the best results by making this choice.

Chapter 8

What Will You Do in the Two-Week Course?

If you want something done, ask a busy person.
—Benjamin Franklin

As I mentioned in chapter 1, weight management is for your health. To maintain good health is a lifelong goal. So is keeping an optimal weight. The two-week-long course outlined below is only a tool, along with your personal and your classmates' experience, to prove that you can "breath yourself thin" as was described in a KAKE TV interview. Bigu Qigong can benefit you as long as you live, if you use it. You will be totally independent in your weight management, as was discussed in the *Wichita Eagle* interview "Qigong Takes, Keeps Her Extra Weight Off."

In this two-week course, you will practice concentrating on the exercise and not letting your mind wander. You will learn how to do it correctly. You will start the consistent practice you need to be the most successful. You will attend class for an hour every day, including weekends, for the two-week period. Wear loose-fitting, comfortable clothing. Go with an open mind and health as your goal, of which losing weight is a part.

Bigu Qigong Two-Week Teaching Schedule

Day	Content	Objectives
1	Concepts of Qigong, Bigu, Bigu Qigong, history Qigong exercise 1: hunger control	• Explain the concepts • Practice exercise 1
2	How does Bigu Qigong work? Eating habits Qigong phenomenon	• Explain why Bigu Qigong works • Check on hunger control • List at least three Qigong phenomena
3	What are you working for? Qigong exercise 2: energy collection	• Explain the importance of health • Practice exercise 2
4	Mind: concentration methods (count breaths, hear breathing) Precautions for the Qigong exercise	• List at least one method to help concentration • Know the precautions for the Qigong exercise
5	Mind/mood checkup: peaceful mind (Village Man)	• Explain the effect of a peaceful mind
6	Mind/mood checkup: tolerance (Nine-Yard Ally)	• Explain the effect of a peaceful mind
7	Summary for the week	• Encourage the student and correct mistakes
8	Consistency and correction	• Explain the importance of consistency
9	Energy Level checkup	• Check on energy level
10	The importance of concentration	• Explain the importance of concentration

11	Following the natural law	• Explain the importance of following the natural law
12	The advantages of the Bigu Qigong—compare to other weight management methods	• List at least three advantages of the Bigu Qigong
13	How to go back to normal eating habits	• Explain the physiological changes of the last two weeks and the smooth transition back to normal eating habits
14	Summary	• Discuss your successes and the things that you need to improve

This two-week course uses the facts to prove that you can control your own weight and your own health without costing a fortune. You do have to spend time to do it, and you will have plenty time to do it because you believe that your health is the most important thing in your life.

Chapter 9

What Do Research, the
Newspaper, and TV Say?

It is health that is real wealth and not pieces of gold and silver.
—Mahatma Gandhi

Research Papers:

Bigu and Weight Loss: Qi as a Food Source

Dr. Qizhi Gao, DOM, Dipl. Ac.
Published by *Kung Fu/Qigong Magazine*, November 1998
Presented at the Second World Congress on Qigong
San Francisco, California
November 1997

In the medical literature, obesity is referred to as a "multifactorial disorder." Defined (by the NIH) as a body weight 20 percent or more above "desirable" weight, over one-third of adult Americans are overweight. Perched at the center of chronic disease risk and psychosocial disability for millions of Americans, successful management of obesity offers unique patient care and public health opportunities. If all Americans were to achieve a normal body weight, it has been estimated that there would be a three-year increase in life expectancy, 25 percent less coronary heart disease, and 35 percent less congestive heart failure and stroke.

56

Unfortunately, obesity is also one of the most difficult and frustrating disorders to manage successfully. Considerable effort is expended by primary care providers and patients with little benefit. Using standard treatments in university settings, only 20 percent of patients lose twenty pounds at two-year follow-up while only 5 percent of patients lose forty pounds. This lack of clinical success has created a never-ending demand for new weight loss treatments.

A truly comprehensive program for weight loss mainly includes three parts: reducing caloric intake, exercise, and behavior modification. The key point is reducing caloric intake because change in weight equals caloric intake minus caloric output, according to the first law of thermodynamics. Normally, the purpose of exercise is to increase the caloric output, and the purpose of behavior modification is to limit the caloric intake with self-control.

Based on the above understanding, Bigu Qigong shows its big advantage on weight loss. Bigu translates literally as "avoid [*bi*] the grain [*gu*]." In practice, it reflects the ability to live solely on qi without food. Bigu is a period during which the Qigong practitioner's vital energy transitions from the air one breathes and the essence of food and water to drawing one's sustenance strictly from the qi in the air. For the experienced Qigong practitioner, this is a natural process that occurs when the accumulation of qi reaches a certain level. The ability to sustain normal body functions from qi only is possible with no change in one's daily routine and has no side effects. Some Qigong practitioners can live on the qi without food for a long period of time and, oftentimes, for achieving and sustaining a much higher energy level through the physical and mental discipline of the Bigu exercise. For weight loss, it combines reducing caloric intake, exercise, and behavior modification altogether.

One of the most elusive principles of Qigong is quantifying qi as a vital force. Scientific methods are just beginning to define its nature, objectively supporting what has been experienced very profoundly on a more personal, subjective level. From the broadest viewpoint, everything is a form of energy. Body energy has an anatomy and a physiology uniquely its own, separate from the physical body. Despite the basic difference of air and food in terms of vibratory function and complexity, there is a homeostatic relationship between them in which one acts as a backup system for the other.

Bigu can be found in many ancient Chinese texts, in individual legend, and in exercise methods to experience. Here are a few examples.

A story from *Bao Puzi's Inner Treaties* said that a man named Jian was hunting in the field when he fell into a deep tomb in his early age. He was so hungry. Then he saw a big turtle. Its head moved up and down to swallow the air. Jian was told that a turtle is good at Daoyin—conducting qi. He imitated the turtle's movement. He did not feel hungry anymore until someone saved him one hundred days later. After that, he had the Bigu ability—living on the air without food. Emperor Wei did not believe this and placed Jian in a room without food. One year later, Jian still was full of energy and his face had a normal, healthy color.

Wang Chong *Lun Heng—Dao Xue Pian* from the Eastern Han dynasty stated, "The people who live on qi have longevity. Although they do not eat enough grain, they are still full of energy."

Among the historical relics unearthed from the Han tomb number 3 at Mawangdui, Changsha, Hunan Province, there was a silk book, *On Abandoning Food and Living on Qi*, and a silk painting, *Daoyin Illustrations*, of the early Western Han dynasty period (third century BC). The former is a method of "inducing, promoting, and conducting qi"; the latter displays forty-four colored *Daoyin Illustrations* in which training exercises are painted.

As a Qigong practitioner, I have personally experienced Bigu twice. From July 20, 1993, until August 3, 1993, my daily diet consisted of a cup of juice or an orange. The first three days were the most difficult as I continued to feel hungry. After the three-day adjustment period, I was able to control my appetite and hunger with the Qigong exercise and gradually increased my energy level as well.

During the two-week period, I continued my normal work routine and required less sleep than normal; physically and mentally I felt very comfortable and relaxed. I lost a total of ten pounds in two weeks and have never gained the weight back. I repeated the same process for a two-week period in 1996 with similar results.

In June of 1996, I conducted a two-week weight loss experiment with twelve subjects, most of whom had no previous Qigong experience. Subjects were initially taught two different Qigong exercises: one to control appetite and one to increase energy level. These exercises facilitated the body switching its primary nutrient source from food to qi. Each subject was encouraged to eat and drink only what the body required. Emphasis was placed on the fact that this was not a deprivation study but rather a study to demonstrate the body's ability to derive sustenance from sources other than food and, in the process, promote weight reduction.

At the conclusion of the two-week study, there was a significant mean weight loss of 11.2 pounds (5.06 kilograms) ($p<. 0001$); mean weight loss per day was 0.9 pounds (0.41 kilograms). Energy levels gradually increased over the two-week period with a concomitant reduction of hunger. Food consumption was rated on a six-point scale with a 6 representing three complete meals. Mean food consumption was rated fewer than 2 for all days except day 3 and day 11 (see table 1).

There was a significant increase in energy levels post exercise for nine of the thirteen days (67 percent). Hunger levels were significantly reduced ten of thirteen days (77 percent). Blood pressure did not significantly change between pre- and post-measures.

Ten of the twelve subjects lost a minimum of nine pounds during the fourteen-day experiment; the two subjects who lost less than nine pounds (three pounds and four pounds, respectively), both performed the exercises less frequently and had higher food consumption. All subjects returned to normal eating habits within three days of terminating the exercise. The results were presented at the Third World Conference on Medical Qigong.

Bigu Qigong is a safe and effective method for weight loss, which uses the exercise to reduce caloric intake under self-control; however, for the lay Qigong practitioner, it is necessary to have an experienced teacher to guide them. Bigu is a viable protocol for long-term, sustained weight loss.

TABLE 1: Hunger and Fatigue levels evaluated before and after Qigong exercises and significance of change

DAY	PRE FATIGUE	POST FATIGUE	SIGNIFI CANCE	PRE HUNGER	POST HUNGER	SIGNIFI CANCE	FOOD CONSUMP TION
1	9.6	7.9	*	7.4	5.6	**	1.4
2	9.1	8.8	NS	7.3	7.8	INCREASE	1.7
3	6.4	9.5	INCREASE	7.2	8.2	INCREASE	2.4
4	6.3	7.5	NS	6.1	4.8	NS	1.7
5	8.4	6.3	***	7.1	4.6	***	1.6
6	8.5	6.1	**	6.7	4.6	**	1.5
7	8.8	6.2	**	6.9	4.8	**	1.1
8	7.5	8.2	**	5.5	3.8	**	1.3
9	7.8	6.4	**	5.7	3.7	**	1.5
10	7.3	6.2	**	5.9	4.4	**	1.3
11	6.6	5.1	*	5.5	3.2	*	2.0
12	5.6	4.4	***	5.3	3.3	***	1.8
13	6.3	4.5	***	5.1	3.2	***	1.2

* = significant at p<. 05
** = significant at p<. 01
*** = significant at p<. 001
NS = nonsignificant
INCREASE = hunger or fatigue level increased post exercise

Utilizing the Innate Self-Regulatory and Self-Healing Capacity on Weight Management

Dr. Qizhi Gao, DOM, Dipl. Ac.
Presented at the ISSSEEM Conference in
Boulder, Colorado
June 1999

www.ibreathin.com

Purpose: Utilizing the innate self-regulatory and self-healing capacity on weight management.

"Overweight and obesity, a growing public health problem, affects 97 million American adults—55 percent of the population. These individuals are at increased risk of illness from hypertension, lipid disorders, type 2 diabetes, coronary heart disease, stroke, gallbladder disease, osteoarthritis, sleep apnea and respiratory problems, and certain cancers. The total costs attributable to obesity-related disease approaches $100 billion annually."[4]

The conventional method (the most successful strategies) for weight loss includes calorie reduction, increased physical activity, and behavior therapy designed to improve eating and physical activity habits.

Do our bodies have any ability to help weight management? Through nearly thirty years of Qigong practice and research, the author believes that Bigu Qigong is one of the most effective ways to utilize the innate self-regulatory and self-healing capacity of the human body to control body weight.

Based on the above understanding, Bigu Qigong demonstrates its big advantage on weight loss. Bigu translates literally as "avoid [*bi*] the grain [*gu*]." In practice, it reflects the ability to live solely on qi without food. Bigu is a period during which the Qigong practitioner's vital energy transitions from the air one breathes and the essence of food and water to drawing one's sustenance strictly from the qi in the air. For the experienced Qigong practitioner, this is a natural process that occurs when the accumulation of qi reaches a certain level. The ability to sustain normal body functions from qi only is possible, with no change in one's daily routine, and there are no side effects. Some Qigong practitioners can live on the qi, without food, for a long period of time, oftentimes achieving and sustaining a much higher energy level through the physical and mental discipline of the Bigu exercise. For weight loss, it combines reducing caloric intake, exercise, and behavior modification altogether.

---

4   National Institutes of Health, "First Federal Obesity Clinical Guidelines Released," *NIH News Release* 17 (June 1998).

The number and selection of subjects: seventy-four

In 1996 the author began a personal and small group experiment. Results were presented at the Third World Conference on Medical Qigong, Beijing, China, 1996. In June 1999, a local newspaper reported that one of my weight management class participants had lost over thirty pounds over a six-month period following her attendance in the class. After receiving a number of public requests, the author conducted this experiment with seventy-four participants over a two-week trial during the period of July 6, 1999, and August 31, 1999. The group's ages ranged from twenty-one to eighty-one. There were seven males and sixty-seven females in the study. According to the Federal Obesity Clinical Guideline by NHLBI, NIDDK,[5] individuals were grouped into three categories: Seven subjects were in the normal weight range (BMI < 25), thirty-six subjects were in the overweight range (25 < BMI < 30), and thirty-one subjects were in the obesity range (BMI > 30). None of the subjects had previous Qigong experience.

Research method: Using the Bigu Qigong exercise to utilize the body's self-regulatory and self-healing function.

During the two-week trial, subjects were taught two different Qigong exercises: one to control appetite and one to increase energy levels. Both exercises were experienced in a sitting or lying-down position, using gentle breaths with mind concentration. Additionally, it was recommended that the exercises be accomplished in fifteen-minute intervals prior to the subjects' three daily meals. Two rules were set: (1) eat only when you are hungry and (2) drink only when you are thirsty. There were no food limitations. Class met one hour a day to do the exercise and discuss each subject's concerns.

The exercises facilitated in switching the body's primary nutrient source from food to qi. Special emphasis was placed on advising subjects that this was not a deprivation study but rather a study to demonstrate the

---

5   National Institutes of Health, "First Federal Obesity Clinical Guidelines Released," *NIH News Release* 17 (June 1998).

body's ability to derive sustenance from sources other than food and, in the process, promote weight reduction.

Results/findings: At the conclusion of the two-week study, fifty-eight of seventy-four attended more than ten classes. There was a significant mean weight loss of 5.7, 5.69, and 7.66 pounds for five subjects from the normal weight group, thirty-one from the overweight group, and twenty-two from the obesity group, respectively. Even sixteen of the seventy-four who attended only six of the classes on the average still lost 2.5, 2.6, and 3.44 pounds, two in the normal weight group, five in the overweight group, and nine from the obesity group, respectively.

The subjects each reported a significant increase in energy levels post exercise for nine of the thirteen days. Hunger levels were significantly reduced ten of thirteen days. Blood pressure did not significantly change between pre- and post-measures.

Discussion: "From the broadest viewpoint, everything is a form of energy. Body energy has an anatomy and physiology uniquely its own separate from the physical body. Despite the basic difference of air and food, the two necessities in life, in terms of vibratory function and complexity, there is a homeostatic relationship between them in which one acts as a back-up system for the other."[6]

Can we find the relationship to utilize the self-regulatory and self-healing capacity on weight management? The success of Bigu Qigong exercise on weight management may provide a good example.

Compared with conventional methods, Bigu Qigong offers more advantages for weight management. The exercise controls hunger utilizing the innate self-regulatory and self-healing capacity from the body itself instead of seeking numerous drugs to limit calorie intake, forcing the body to change its own law unwillingly and causing side effects. Additionally, the exercise uses body fat as a source of energy rather than requiring subjects to do different physical exercises to burn

---

6   Qizhi Gao, Qigong and Weight Loss, "Qi as a Food Source," in *Third World Conference on Medical Qigong*, (Beijing, China, 1996): 144.

up the fat. Many exercises are not fit for all ages, and body weight is regained when physical exercise is stopped. As a behavior therapy designed to improve eating and physical activity habits, the exercise offered a solid base to ensure subjects were not hungry and were full of energy, thus assisting them in following the two rules: eat and drink only when needed.

Mind concentration in conjunction with the special breathing patterns used in Bigu Qigong played an important role in achieving study results, that is, digestive function stimulation, heart and lung circulation, and increased circulation to the head and face, all of which are key in achieving optimum self-regulation and self-healing.

During the first five days of the study, one subject was unable to concentrate due to family issues. The subject lost no weight. Once the author consulted with the subject, her concentration improved, and she lost six pounds during the remaining nine days of the study.

Attendance was also a key in achieving the subjects' weight-loss goals.

Summary: Bigu Qigong is a safe and effective method for weight loss, which uses the exercise to reduce caloric intake under self-control; however, for the lay Qigong practitioner, it is necessary to have an experienced teacher to guide them. Bigu is a viable protocol for long-term, sustained weight loss.

Newspaper Article:

Qigong Takes, Keeps Her Extra Weight off
The Wichita Eagle main edition
Tuesday, June 29, 1999, page 1B
Living section, It Worked for Me column
Copyright (c) 1999, The Wichita Eagle & Beacon Publishing Co.

Name: Sylvia Gorup, Wichita.
Personal: 48; married; two grown children; title officer at Security Abstract and Title.

Problem: Extra weight that "just kind of creeps on as you get older." Gorup had dieted and regained weight several times through the years. She had been exercising five days a week and "kind of watched what I was eating, but not really," but hadn't seen any change in her weight.

What she did: Enrolled in a Qigong (chee-gong) weight management class at Evergreen Wellness Center, a Traditional Chinese Medicine clinic in Wichita. Lost 30 pounds in about five months and has kept the weight off.

How she did it: Qigong emphasizes breathing, meditation and stationary and moving exercises to enhance the flow of energy through the body. Gorup started a 30-day exercise class with a friend who was seeking relief for fibromyalgia. During the class, teacher Qizhi Gao talked about using Qigong for weight loss; class members talked him into offering the weight loss class.

The class, which met for an hour every day for two weeks (including weekends), taught Gorup to "eat when you're hungry and drink when you're thirsty" and breathe in a specific way that pushes the diaphragm up and gives her a feeling of fullness. She also learned an "energy-gathering" meditation. The breathing exercises and meditation are to be done three times a day, for 20 to 30 minutes a time. "You got down to the point where you ate hardly anything, but yet you weren't hungry and weren't tired," says Gorup, who says she was skeptical going into the class but tried to remain open-minded.

She lost 18 pounds during the two weeks and continued to lose afterward; weight loss among class members ranged from five to 22 pounds. Gorup ate what she wanted but found that she could no longer easily digest some foods.

Because she could eat what she wanted, she felt no sense of denial. She took the class again earlier this year, along with three co-workers. This time, she lost four or five pounds; the co-workers lost about 10 pounds each. She hasn't regained any of the weight. Her hints for success: "Part of it is buying into the philosophy" of Chinese medicine, she says. "You've got to want to do it." Take the class with a partner "to motivate each other." The diet was easy for her because "you didn't have to think about what you were eating, you didn't have to think about weighing your food." Class members kept daily records of what they ate and how they felt, physically and emotionally. . . .

Television interview:

Breathing Yourself Thin
Are you trying to shed some extra pounds this New Year? Tired of going to the gym or starving yourself to lose weight?

Jemelle Holopirek
KAKE News at 10pm
KAKE, February 3, 2011

Are you trying to shed some extra pounds this New Year?

Tired of going to the gym or starving yourself to lose weight?

Most people exercise, run, lift weights to lose weight. But now some say forget that. They are doing something that's called Qigong (CHEE-GUNG).

"I will try anything I'm kind of desperate at this time."

Brandy Brinkley is a mother of two and she's tried dozens of diets, but nothing's worked.

"I hope to get more healthy and I would like to lose 20 pounds"

Qigong has been a part of Chinese medicine for more than 2000 years, and now it's being used in the United States for weight management.

"Sitting there and special breathing and certain mind setting and they will lose weight."

Dr. Qizhi Gao teaches Qigong at his East Wichita office. It's a 14-day program with an hour-long class every night.

www.ibreathin.com

The method involves breathing, positioning of your body and mental focus.

These techniques should be performed before each meal.

"The people will not feel like eating, and they will not feel much hungry."

There are two rules: eat when you're hungry, and drink when you're thirsty. This may sound easier than it is.

"I kept thinking am I thirsty and I couldn't really figure it out. I think I just eat all the time and I think it will help to take a time out before I eat."

At the end of the 14-day program, the class had dropped from 17 members to 10. Many found it hard to commit to class every night, but the people who stuck with the program saw results.

"Well I've lost almost 10 pounds in 14 days, really exciting because I didn't work out and I ate the same food as I would prior to coming here."

Madeline Norland also liked the number on the scale.

"I lost 6.7, nearly 7 pounds, which is nice to see over 14 days."

As a whole, the 10-member class lost nearly 60 pounds.

"I did eat less, the breathing exercise really taught us to suppress our appetite."

"It's something I plan to do the rest of my life."

Dr. Gao says Qigong is like exercising in the fact that you have to be consistent, you should do the breathing techniques three times a day, about 15–30 minutes before you eat a meal.

Printed in the United States
By Bookmasters